ESSENTIAL OIL FOR HEALTHY LIFE

THE COMPLETE USER GUIDE TO
ESSENTIAL OIL + HEALTH BENEFITS

JAMES AMELIA

Copy Right© 2019
James Amelia

This publication may not be reproduced, distributed or transmitted by any means without the prior written consent of the author first had and obtained. The facts herein provided is truthful in all its entirety and coherent, in that no legal responsibility, in the form of consideration or else by the use or misuse of any strategies, procedures or directions contained within shall lie against the author such liability thereon is the sole and the utter obligation of the reader solely. Under no situation will any legal duty or blames be imputed or held out unfavorable the publisher(s) for any form of compensation, damages, pecuniary loss due to the information contained herein be it direct or indirect.

The information offered here is for the purposes of information only and is universal as such. The information presented here is without any form of contract or guarantee or indemnity whether with the reader or any third party.

TABLE OF CONTENTS

COCONUT OIL 1

HEALTH USES OF COCONUT OIL 2

HOW TO MAKE COCONUT OIL 10

HOME USES OF COCONUT OIL 24

TEA TREE OIL 37

CHAPTER FIVE 39

THE BENEFITS OF TEA TREE OIL 39
HOW TO USE TEA TREE OIL FOR DANDRUFF
TREATMENT 40
TTO AS NATURAL MOISTURIZERS 41
HOW TO USE TTO 42
HOW TO USE TTO TO TREAT HEAD LICE 44
TREATMENT OF ACNE WITH TEA TREE OIL 45
HOW TO USE TTO IN TREATING ACNE 45

How to use TTO to Treat Eczema and psoriasis 46

How to use TTO 47

Effective Means of Controlling Gland that produces Skin Oil... 48

How to use TTO to Treat Stye 49

How to use Tea Tree Oil for the Treatment of Belly Button Infections 50

How to use TTO to Heal/Dry socket pains 50

How to Prepare and Use TTO to Control Body Odour 51

How to use Tea Tree oil as Room Spray 52

CHAPTER SIX 53

You Can Make TTO At Home 53

CHAPTER SEVEN 55

Tips and Tricks for Using TTO 55
Dosages of Tea Tree Oil................................... 57
Side effects of Tea Tree Oil.............................. 58
How to Buy Tea Tree Oil Online 59

CHAPTER ONE

COCONUT OIL

Coconut oil is an edible oil that is extracted from the meats of a matured coconuts harvested from coconut palm. Coconut oil benefits in several way which includes; skin care, weight loss, improving digestion, hair care, treating yeast infections, and boosting immunity against a host of infections and diseases. Coconut oil is not only used in tropical countries, where coconut plantations are abundant, but also in the United States, Canada, Australia and Europe. Day by day, people are discovering the wonders of this oil and it is thereby gaining more popularity throughout the world.

More than 90% of coconut oil consists of saturated fats (this is not to scar you and It is not as bad as it sounds), along with traces of a few unsaturated fatty acids, such as monounsaturated fatty acids and polyunsaturated fatty acids. Most of the saturated fatty acids are medium chain triglycerides, which are supposed to assimilate well in the body systems.

HEALTH USES OF COCONUT OIL

There exist several health benefits coconut oil usage, the most important ones being its usefulness in skin care and hair care.

Skin Care

Coconut oil is an effective moisturizer and excellent massage oil for all types of skin, including dry skin. There is no adverse side effects on the skin from the application of this oil unlike other mineral oil. Coconut oil has been safely used for thousands of years for flaking and preventing dryness of skin. The usage of coconut oil could be considered as a recent fad, although it has been around for ages.

Coconut oil helps in the treatment of various skin problems, including psoriasis, eczema, dermatitis, and other skin infections. This is why, coconut oil forms the main ingredient of various body care products like lotions, creams and soaps that are used for skin care. Also, coconut oil delays the appearance of wrinkles and sagging of skin, which are majorly associated with aging. The recognition to this benefit goes to her well-known antioxidant properties.

<u>Hair Care</u>

Women in the tropical coastal regions of the world with long and shining hairs uses coconut oil for their hair almost daily. This is the reason for their long and shining hairs. This coconut oil helps in a healthy hair growth and gives a shine to those strands. Coconut oil is also very effective in reducing protein loss, which if you do not check it, could lead to various unhealthy qualities in your hair. This is why coconut oil is used as a hair care oil, and also used in the in the manufacturing of various conditioners and dandruff relief creams that we have today. To use coconut oil, apply it topically to your hair or use a coconut oil hair mask for your hair directly.

Coconut oil is an excellent conditioner and helps the re-growth process of damaged hair. Also, Coconut oil provides the essential proteins that is needed for nourishing and healing damaged hair. Research has shown that Coconut oil provides better protection to hair from damage caused by hygral fatigue.

By using coconut oil regularly, massaging your head with it, you can be rest assured that your scalp is dandruff free, even when your scalp is chronically dry. Also, Coconut oil helps in keeping your hair and scalp free from lice and lice eggs (although this is not common).

Weight Loss

Coconut oil contains short and medium-chain fatty acids which helps in shedding off excessive weight. Research has shown that Coconut oil helps to reduce abdominal obesity in women. Also, Coconut oil is easy to digest when compared to other edible oils and also helps in healthy functioning of the thyroid and endocrine system. Furthermore, Coconut oil increases the metabolic rate of the body by removing stress on the pancreas, thereby, burning more calories and helping overweight and obese people lose weight. People living in the tropical coastal areas, that uses coconut oil on a daily basis as their primary cooking oil, are usually not fat, overweight or obese. Many persons today focus on exercises in order to lose weight, ranging from using indoor machines to outdoor exercises like running and doing other sports. In as much as this is a good approach to weight loss, adding other products like coconut oil enhances your weight loss efforts faster.

Dental Care

One of the essential component of our teeth is Calcium and since coconut oil helps in the absorption of calcium by the body, it helps in the development of a very strong teeth. Coconut oil also helps to prevent tooth decay. A recent study suggests that Coconut oil is also beneficial in reducing plaque formation and plaque-induced gingivitis.

Improves Immunity

Coconut oil is very good in improving your body immunity. Coconut oil strengthens your immune system this because Coconut oil contains antimicrobial lipids, caprylic acid, lauric acid, and capric acid, which have antibacterial, antiviral and antifungal properties. The human body converts lauric acid into monolaurin, which studies has shown to be an effective way to deal with viruses and bacteria that cause diseases like influenza, herpes, cytomegalovirus, and also HIV. This unique oil helps in fighting harmful bacteria like Helicobacter pylori and Listeria monocytogenes and other harmful protozoa {for instance Giardia lamblia}.

Boosts Digestion

This wonder oil helps to improve the digestive system, and thus, prevents different stomach and digestion-related problems which includes irritable bowel syndrome (IBS). The saturated fats present in coconut oil have an antimicrobial properties that helps in dealing with different bacteria, fungi, and parasites that may cause indigestion. Coconut oil also helps in the absorption of other nutrients such as vitamins, minerals, and amino acids.

Prevents Candida

Candida is also known as systemic candidiasis and this is a tragic disease that is caused by an excessive and uncontrolled growth of yeast called Candida albicans in your stomach region. Coconut oil therefore provides a relief from the inflammation that is caused by candida, which is both internally and externally. Coconut oil's high moisture retaining capacity keeps the skin from cracking or peeling off. Caprylic acid, lauric acid, caproic acid, Capric acid, and myristic acid found in coconut oil help in eliminating Candida albicans.

Unlike other pharmaceutical used for candida treatments, the effect of coconut oil is gradual and not sudden or drastic, which gives the patient enough time to get used to the withdrawal symptoms or Herxheimer reactions. In the treatment of this condition, it is better that people should gradually and systematically increase their intakes of coconut oil, and should not from the onset start with a large quantity of the oil.

Keeping Organs Healthy

The availability of a medium chain triglycerides and fatty acids that is present in coconut oil helps in preventing liver diseases. This is because triglycerides and fatty are easily converted into energy when they gets to the liver, thereby reducing the liver's workload and also preventing accumulation of fat in the live. Also, Coconut oil helps in preventing gall bladder and kidney diseases and it helps to dissolve kidney stones. Coconut oil is also said to be useful in keeping the pancreas healthy by treating pancreatitis in the body.

Speeds Up Healing

When coconut oil are applied to infected areas, it forms a chemical layer that protects the infected body part from external dust, fungi, air, bacteria, and viruses. Coconut oil are highly effective on bruises because it speeds up the healing process of damaged tissues of your body.

According to the Coconut Research Center, coconut oil kills the viruses that cause influenza, herpes, hepatitis, measles, SARS, and other serious health risks. Coconut oil also kills bacteria that cause throat infections, ulcers, urinary tract infections, gonorrhea, and pneumonia. Also, coconut oil is effective in the elimination of all fungi and yeast that cause ringworm, diaper rash, thrush and athlete's foot.

CHAPTER TWO

HOW TO MAKE COCONUT OIL

Step 1:

Get a matured brown coconuts

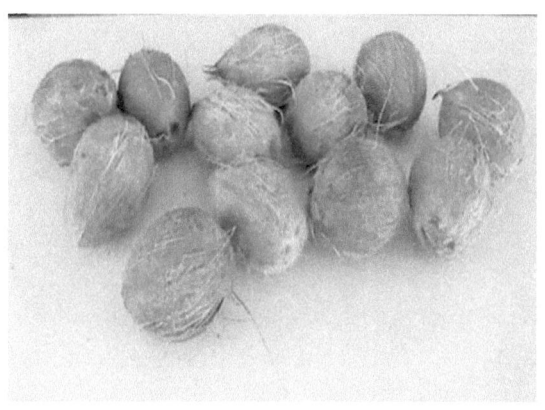

The first step in making your own coconut oil is for you to get a brown coconuts mature at any grocery store near you. Ensure that the coconut is matured enough and your coconut meats is strong and edible.

The number of coconuts that you have depends on the quantity of oil that you desire to make. If you want coconut oil, you have to increase the number of coconuts and yield also depends on the size, quality and freshness of the coconuts. The greater the coconuts, the higher yield will have. Five to six coconuts can yield one cup of oil.

Step 2

Open your coconuts

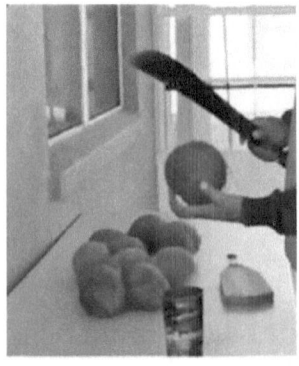

To open your coconut, you first of all put a bowl under your coconuts to collect the water from the coconuts or do it over a sink. In opening the coconut, hold it in one hand and use your hammer or back of the cleaver to sharply tap the center of the coconut against the grain. Do this repeatedly until the coconut shell cleave open. Strain the water from the coconut and keep it so it can be used later on to extract your coconut milk.

I suggest that you empty your bowl before opening your next coconut should in case the coconut is bad. Discard bad coconuts, they smell rancid and their meat can be runny, slimy, and gross. Coconuts that are good do not smell and their meat are hard and white and they are the perfect coconuts for making coconut oil.

Step 3

Remove the coconut meat

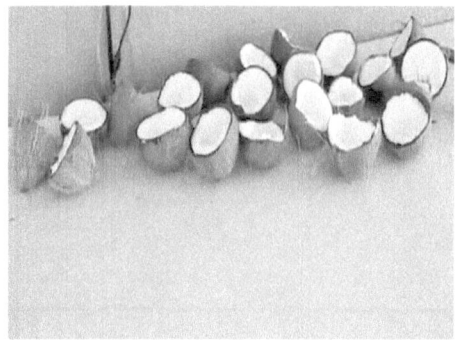

In order to remove your coconut meat, you will have to use the hammer or cleaver and a sturdy knife. Gently tap the shell of the coconut in order to remove the back using your cleaver or hammer. In most cases, the coconut shell will pop right out and if the shell does not pop out, then you have to insert the sturdy knife between the meat and shell and slightly twist it.

Know that the coconut shells can be unstable sometimes and you have to be very careful when tapping and using the knife so you don't injure yourself. Dispose the coconut shells or use them to make cute decorations or you can as well add the smaller pieces to your garden.

Step 4

Grate or shred the coconut meat

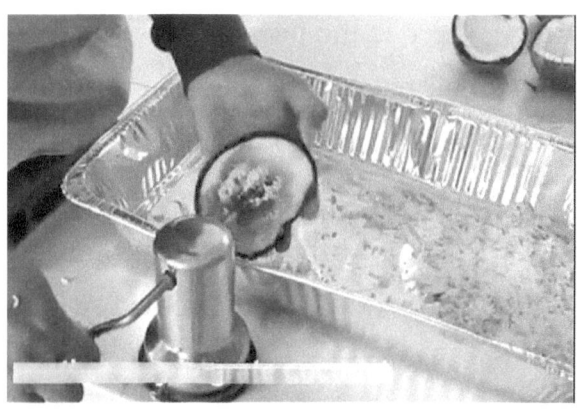

If you are using electric or manual coconut scrapers, you can shred your coconut meat directly from the coconut shell. Make sure that you place a bowl under the scrapers just to collect all the gratings. Should in case you do not have these scrapers, you can use the rough side of the grater to shred your extracted coconut meat. This can take a little while to get it done and if are not careful, you can accidentally grate your finger, but it is however one of the finest way to get coconut meat into a really fine consistency.

However in order to save your fingers and to save time, you can use a blender or a food processor. In this method, there is the need to cut your coconut meats into small pieces to make it easier for your appliances. There may also be need to add water just to be sure that your coconut meat blends properly. By adding water to your coconut pieces inside your blender, the end product will be a slurry-like consistency.

Step 5

Extract your coconut milk

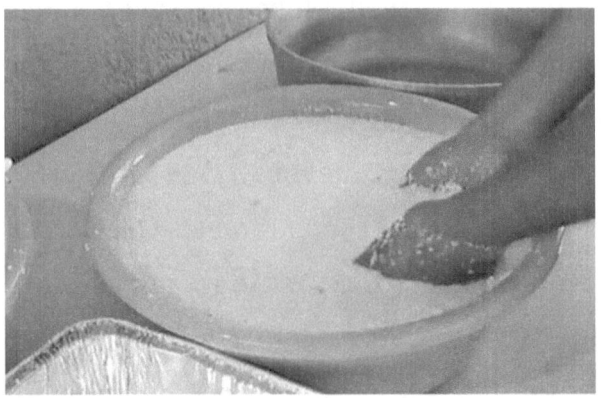

Use the juicer to extract your coconut milk. Load the chute with your grated coconut meat and switch the appliance on. Your coconut milk pours out right and while your coconut meat left is dry. You can as well add your coconut meat slurry from your blender to the juicer. To double your juice, collect the dry coconut meat, mix them with a little water and then add it back to the chute again.

Should in case you don't have a juicer, there is no need to worry, all you need do is to add a little water to your grated/shredded coconut and squeeze your coconut meat. The water will start turning white, that's your coconut milk. The more you squeeze your coconut meat, the more the milk you will get out.

The slurry can also be work from your blender using the same method.

Step 6

Strain your coconut milk

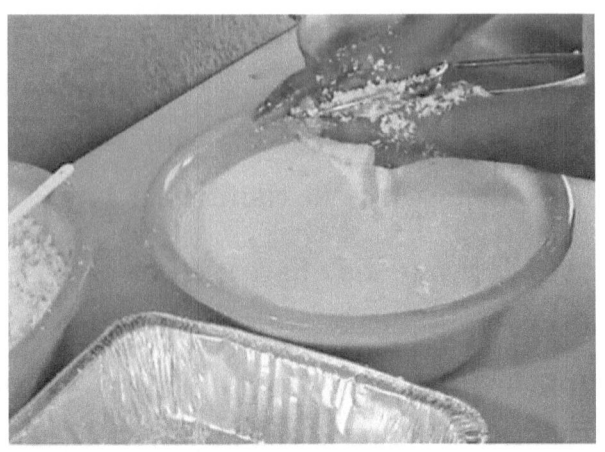

At this step, you will require a strainer, or cheesecloth or any clean cloth. Your coconut milk and meat from your blender, gratings, or juicer must be properly strained to in order to remove particles from your coconut milk. If necessary, you can double strain and triple strain. Ensure that you squeezed out as much milk as possible from your coconut meat.

If you like you can eat the coconut meat that is left behind or you can as well add it to your garden as an all-natural fertilizer. It is a great source of fiber.

Step 7

Allow the coconut milk to sit overnight

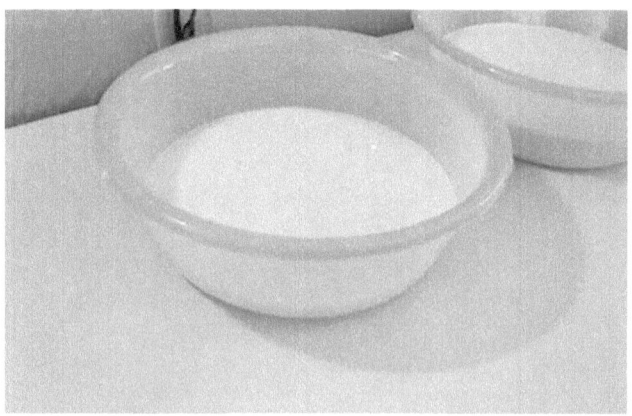

When you are very certain that your coconut milk is properly strained, place the coconut milk in a large bowl and leave it sit undisturbed in a cool place over the night. You can put it in the fridge to ensure that it stays cool throughout the night. If it is warm, your milk will start to smell a little rancid and the odour will then transfer to the oil. It is therefore important to keep your milk in a cool place overnight. You can as well cover the milk with a thin cloth while leaving it overnight.

Step 8

Scoop out cold-pressed, virgin coconut oil

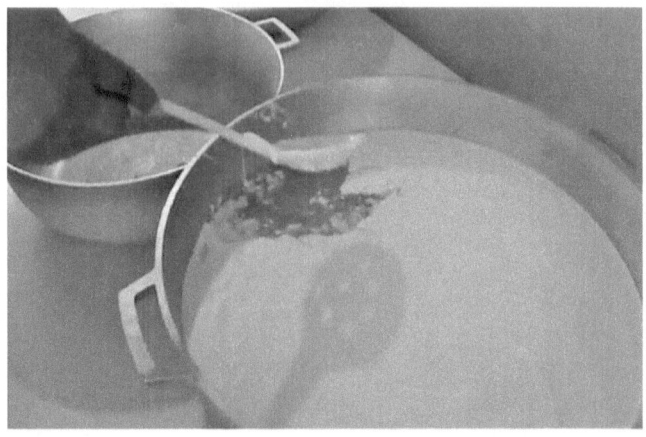

In the morning, you will discover that your coconut milk has separated into a solid, white layer on top of your bowl and clear-ish liquid underneath. Gently remove the solid white layer using a spoon. It is your cold-pressed, extra virgin coconut oil and is also called coconut curd or coconut cream.

You will observe that your oil will have a slight watery feel to it. The reason for this is because there is still water available in your oil layer. With time, the water will dry out. You can put the oil in a bottle and store it in a cool place or in the fridge. Once your oil is stored in a cool place, it will be good for several months even upto a year.

Step 9

Heat the coconut curd

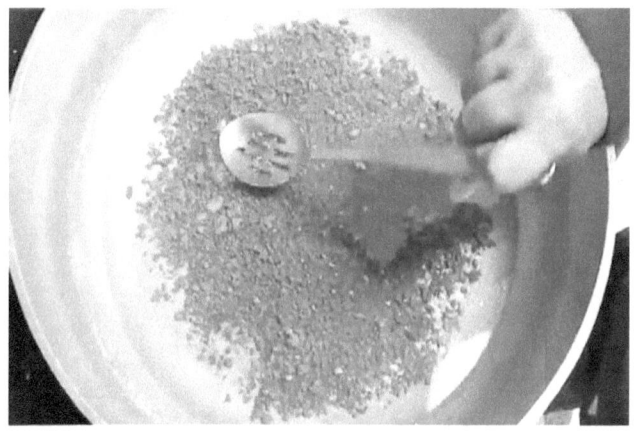

To make it a pure coconut oil, there is the need to further process the cold-pressed, coconut curd/virgin coconut oil to remove the excess water. In doing this, add your coconut curd to a heavy-bottomed pot over medium heat. Make sure you stir continuously in order to prevent the curd from sticking. In about 10 – 15 minutes, you will notice that the curd will separate into light colored oil and white particles. Within the next few minutes, you will see that your oil has changes to a pale yellow colour and the particles become brown. At this point you can turn off the heat.

Step 10

Strain your coconut oil

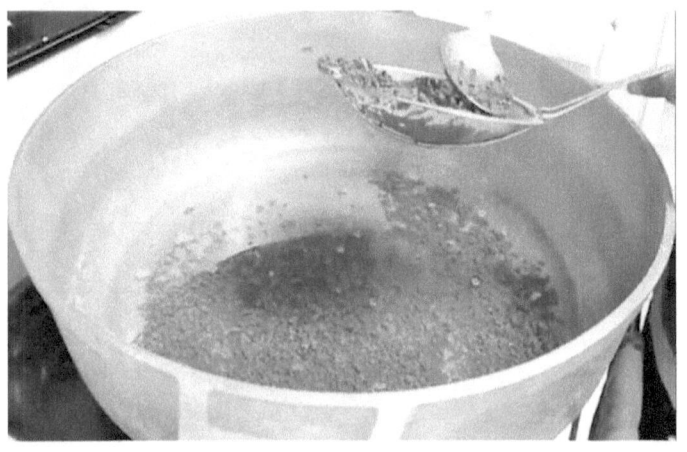

Carefully strain your oil while it is still hot, using a cheesecloth or any other type of cloth. You may find tiny brown specks settling in the oil if you don't strain it.

Step 11

Extract your oil as much as possible

Your brown curd particles also contain a lot of oil and it is therefore a good idea for you to squeeze as much oil as possible out of them. Carefully do this while they are still hot because if they get cold, the oil in them will solidify around the particles and you won't be able to get them out.

You can therefore strain your hot curd particles using few methods, for example, you can twist your cheese cloth to its ends and keep on twisting until some oil come out of it. Also, you can place your cheese cloth on a slotted spoon, and squeeze down on your cloth using something heavy or another spoon. Be careful to get as much oil as you can out without getting burned.

What you get as final products are 100% pure coconut oil and brown curd particles. If you use 3 big sized coconuts, you will get approximately 90 milliliters of coconut oil. When this oil are stored and kept in cool conditions, the oil will turn white and last for months or even up to a year. You can use this pure coconut oil for oil pulling and cooking and also it is great for all your skin care and beauty regimes.

CHAPTER THREE

HOME USES OF COCONUT OIL

The uses of coconut oil are broken into four different categories: Household, Body and Skin Care, Natural Medicine, and Food Uses.

<u>Coconut Oil Food Uses</u>

1. "Buttering Your Toast": Try spreading coconut oil on your sprouted grain bread, for breakfast in the morning instead of the conventional butter. That slight coconut flavor that comes out of especially an unrefined coconut oils, gives a lovely taste and aroma to your toast.
2. Sautéing and Frying: Coconut oil is great for your cooking at a high heat because of their high smoke point. Several other oils for instance the olive oil can oxidize when heated and since coconut oil is made up of healthy saturated fats, the oil remains stable under high temperatures.

3. Creamer for Your Coffee: when you add a spoonful of coconut oil to your coffee, this gives you an extra boost of energy and replace dairy creamer. When you put your hot coffee in a blender, with your coconut oil and the natural sweetener that you desire, and blend, without adding any dairy, you will be surprised at the rich creamy flavor.
4. Natural Energy Booster: The medium chain triglycerides available in coconut oil, when combined with chia seeds, will boost your energy when you need a mid-afternoon pickup, or after a strenuous exercise. Chia seeds are well known for their ability to boost performance, and endurance while your coconut oil aids in digestion and metabolizing of your chia seeds. Combine 1 tablespoon of your coconut oil with ½ tablespoon of chia seeds, and enjoy from your spoon, or spread on sprouted grain bread.

5. Boost Nutrients in Smoothies: adding 1 - 2 tablespoons of your coconut oil to any fruit smoothie form a boost of cholesterol fighting compounds. This however improves the texture and mouth feel of smoothies, while adding to your diet healthy fats.
6. Topping for Baked Potatoes: you can add coconut oil to your baked sweet potatoes instead of the conventional butter and then sprinkle on cinnamon. It can also be used for baked sweet potato French fries adding some rosemary and sea salt.
7. Sports Drink Replacement: this wonder oil gives to your body quick energy in the form of its quick acting MCFA fats. In place of sugary processed drinks, you can add coconut oil and chia seeds to water with fresh fruit for energy boost.
8. Prolong the Freshness of Eggs: coconut oil can be used to seal the pores in an egg shell and can also prolong the life of the eggs in your refrigerator. Rob a small amount of

coconut oil over the shells of your eggs and allow it to penetrate, which will help prevent exposure to oxygen. Doing this, should be able extend the life of your eggs for about 1 to 2 weeks.

9. Natural Throat Lozenge: coconut oil can be used instead of store bought lozenges that are usually made using artificial colors and flavors. Swallowing 1 teaspoon of coconut oil about 2 to 3 times in a day can help to ease the pain of a sore throat or cough, and you combine coconut oil with licorice root tea for a natural throat soother.

10. Coconut oil Replace Unhealthy Fats for Baking: it is possible for you bake with coconut oil. You can make use of the same amount as your vegetable oil or butter that is called for in your recipe. Coconut oil can be used to grease cake pans and baking sheets, and your baked cakes will simply slide right out.

Coconut Oil Beauty & Skin Uses

11. Coconut oil helps in Wrinkle Reduction: A touch of coconut oil in areas of concern around eyes, and under the eyes to help fight pre-maturing aging. Let the oil on stay overnight in order to soak in, and wake up looking refreshed. Coconut oil also to help remove those dark circles around the eyes. When coconut is mixed with frankincense oil, it has additional benefits for anti-aging.

12. Coconut oil Lock in Moisture After Showers: Coconut oil helps in hydrating dry skin and also helps to soothe skin after shaving. Apply coconut oil liberally after your shower all over your body. Also, coconut oil has a natural SPF as part of it component and this is great for protecting your skin from sun damage.

13. Coconut oil for Natural Skin Moisturizer: when you use coconut oil for skin health, it works well as a moisturizer for your face.

Coconut oil absorbs quickly and it is non-greasy when applied to the body. Coconut is a solid at room temperature but this same oil melts quickly when it comes into contact with hands.

14. Coconut oil for Natural Makeup Remover: A very small quantity of coconut oil is enough to quickly liquefy your eye makeup, making the eye makeup easy to be wiped off. Ensure that the coconut oil is rubbed gently in the upper lids and the lower lids in a circular motion after which you wipe it off using a warm cloth. The edge that coconut oil have over commercial eye makeup removers is that when used, coconut oil will not irritate or sting eyes and its also help to hydrate roundabout the eyes when applied.

15. Coconut oil for Homemade Toothpaste: equally mix parts of coconut oil and your baking soda and mix in a few drops of peppermint essential oil to have your homemade toothpaste ready for use.

16. Coconut oil for Insect Repellent: to use coconut oil as an insect repellent, you have to add a tablespoon of coconut oil with some couple of drops of peppermint, tea tree oil and rosemary to repel mosquitos, flies, bees and gnats. Using this, is a safe alternative to DEET and this can be applied safely on all areas of the body.
17. Coconut oil for Personal Lubricant: the use of coconut oil for personal lubricant is very safe and effective. Compared with commercial preparations, coconut oil is antibacterial, antifungal and antimicrobial properties which helps to keep the vaginal flora healthy.
18. Coconut oil for Cellulite Solution: do you want to fight stubborn and unsightly cellulite? Then add 1 tablespoon of coconut oil to 10 drops of grapefruit essential oil and massage into affected areas in a firm circular motion.

19. Coconut oil helps Prevent and Treat Dandruff: Coconut oil help you to get rid of dandruff and also help to encourage new hair growth. After application, rinse again and again and then style as you use to. Once you have done this, your hair would be healthy, shiny and full of body. Should in case the coconut oil weighs down your hair, it is advisable you use less amount next time and you ensure rinse well until clean.
20. Coconut oil for Massage Oil: this is a soothing and conditioning massage oil. Put a couple of drops of peppermint oil and lavender oil to help heal sore muscles and stimulate relaxation of the mind.
21. Coconut oil for Anti-Fungal Cream: Given to her antibiotic capabilities, coconut oil can be used to treat skin fungus and athletes foot. To do this, apply some quantity of coconut to the affected area and when you have done this, you can either leave the oil on or you can

wipe off with a towel after that the coconut oil has set in for a reasonable time.

Coconut Oil Household Uses

22. Coconut oil Remove Gum From Furniture or Hair: Apply coconut oil to help you remove gum easily if you have ever had gum stuck in your hair or on your coach, without leaving any stains or colors.
23. Carrier Oil for Essential Oil Diffuser: In place of candles that contain artificial scents and chemicals, coconut oil used with essential oils in an essential oil diffuser in your home.
24. Coconut oil for Laundry Detergent: mix your coconut oil with lye, essential oils and water to create a non-toxic soapy liquid which is perfect for cleaning your clothes. This method will have a negative effects on your fabric or not irritate your skin, like many other detergents do. This is a great solution

for those prone to allergies and sensitive skin.

25. Coconut oil Prevent Dust: Using little quantity of coconut oil on the surfaces materials like plastic, wood or cement that tend to gather dust helps to mitigate the dust. Take a little amount of your oil and rub over the area and while you allow it to dry. There is no need to wash off the coconut oil since it is antibacterial and antifungal.

26. Coconut oil for Furniture Polish: Coconut oil is essential and can be used on wood, metal surfaces and granite counter tops to give your furniture a shiny look. Also, this will assist to cover up scratches, reduce dusk and clean your furniture and home surfaces, as well.

Coconut Oil Medicinal Uses

27. Coconut Oil Boost Immunity: The unique nutritional profile of coconut oil that is rich with capric acid, caprylic acid and lauric acid

provides for strong antifungal, antibacterial, antimicrobial and antiviral properties that is imbedded with an immune boosting effect. These properties of coconut oil helps fighting those foreign elements that is present in the body, and your immune system is better equipped to respond properly when attacked by foreign antibodies.

28. Coconut Oil for Alzheimer's Treatment and Brain Health Protector: Several studies has tried to attribute that coconut oil may be an effective natural treatment for Alzheimer's disease. At the moment, the studies of coconut for Alzheimer's treatment is premature inconclusive.

29. Coconut Oil Help Fight Inflammation: According to a research carried out, virgin coconut oil that is well prepared without high-heat or chemical treatment, tends to exhibits an inhibitory effect on chronic inflammation. Coconut oil also supports

both a healthy liver and kidneys. This study however supports the regular intakes of virgin coconut oil to help fight inflammation since inflammation is one of the common cause of many chronic diseases today.

30. Coconut Oil Help Fight Heart Disease: Coconut oil has been vilified for decades of due to its saturated fat content, however modern researches are now showing that a medium-chain fatty acids and coconut oil are beneficial to the health of the heart and also help regulate high blood pressure.

31. Coconut Oil Help Balance Cholesterol Levels: The triglycerides and fats in coconut oil have been shown to increase HDL cholesterol and lower LDL cholesterol, in other words supporting heart health. According to a study 2015 that examined coronary artery disease patients, "coconut oil consumption helped increase HDL cholesterol and also reduced waist circumference".

CHAPTER FOUR

TEA TREE OIL

Melaleuea alternitolia, a rich source of Tea Tree Oil (TTO for short and whenever I refer to this short abbreviation in this book, I am referring to tea tree oil), a native of New South Wales and Queensland, Australia, it has become so popular today due to its versatile usage. Tea Tree Oil is also an essential oil that possesses very virile antibacterial properties and can treat many infections.

The Aboriginals have employed the use of TTO as medicine for many centuries. The leaves are pulverised by the aborigines and the oil extracted which is mostly inhaled for the treatment of coughs, cold, and skin related diseases.

At present, tea tree oil is used today as one hundred percent undiluted or clean oil. There are also diluted forms of TTO which are in use today.

Tea Tree Essential Oil Contents

The first compound that is found in TTO is terpinen 4 01, which has been proven to destroy fungi, bacteria, and some types of viruses. Surprisingly, terpinen 4 ol, has been known to raise the activity of white blood cells which also helps in fighting germs and other alien invaders. As a result of this anti-germs property which TTO possess, it has become very valuable in the treatment of many skin related conditions and infections.

Tea Tree Oil: It How Does work?

Tea tree oil can be termed an essential oil with fresh camphor smell. Derived from the leaves of Melaleuca alternifolia, commonly found in Queensland and New South Wales, Australia. Its tree grows up to 7 meters tall.

The question whether this oil work is important. One reason why the Tea tree oil works is because of its structure and composition. The oil has over 100 components, but the major elements are sesquiterpenes, monoterpenes, and their individual alcohols.

Benefits of Tea Tree Oil

It has been explained above that TTO has multifarious uses to which the oil can be effectively used for. We will consider some of these uses for skin, hair and for other purposes.

CHAPTER FIVE

THE BENEFITS OF TEA TREE OIL
Thicker and Longer Hair

If your hair is short, and you experience frequent breakage of your hair, I present to you your ultimate solution – Tea Tree Oil. Tea Tree Oil can enhance the growth of your hair by unclogging hair follicles and provide nourishment for hair root.

How to use TTO for Longer and Thicker Hair

To use Tea Tree Oil for the purposes of making your hair thicker and stronger, simply apply the oil to your hair by spraying it. Fill your bottle of glass spray with enough quantity of water and add 5 drops of TTO for every ounce. Then spray it in the morning and allow it throughout the day for hair growth.

Effective Remedy for Dandruff

Due to the high presence of antibacterial and fungi properties, TTO is ideal for the treating of dandruff. The Tea tree oil battles the fungi that cause dandruff without necessarily drying your hair scalp. Besides it ability to kill dandruff, TTO serves as a good natural conditioner that prevents issues that causes scalp flake

How to use Tea Tree Oil for Dandruff Treatment

If you want to treat dandruff with TTO, add normal shampoo to hair approximately ten drops for every eight ounces of shampoo. Before washing your hair, make sure that you allow the shampoo and the TTO to mix well for at least 5 minutes. If you desire faster and quicker results from the use of TTO for the treatment of dandruff, use it overnight. Just add a ¾ bottle of olive oil, almond oil, coconut oil, jojoba oil, etc. After that, add 15 drops of TTO and blend it. Apply it to your hair scalp and massage it for some few minutes and ensure that your scalp is wholly saturated.

TTO as Natural Moisturizers

Tea Tree oil has amazing benefits because of its ability to nourish and moisturize your dry scalp. It clears any blockage in your pores and prevents dry hair.

How to use TTO as Moisturizers

Mix a few droplets of jojoba oil with TTO and massage the mix for about 15 minutes. Rinse it very well and wash your hair. Carry out this process as regularly as you can. It can also stop itchy hair. Add shampoo to your hair and add a few droplets of your normal hair conditioner. Blend it well and add it to your scalp. Allow it some few minutes before washing.

Hair Cleanser

Tea Tree oil performs various hair functions. It can be used as your regular shampoo at home for your hair.

How to use Tea Tree oil as your hair cleanser

Add some few droplets of Tea Tree oil to your normal shampoo. By doing so, it gives your shampoo added therapeutic elements. Apply the mix to your hair scalp and massage it for some time. After that, rinse it very well.

Treating Dry and Itchy Hair

This is another amazing benefit of using Tea Tree oil for your hair. It can be used to treat dry and itchy hair. You will need any carrier, that is, any oil of your choice such as jojoba oil, almond oil, or sesame oil. Since Tea tree oil destroys microbes that are known for causing damage to the scalp, it calms your itchy scalp and subsequently heals it. The common causes of itchiness are dirty scalp, dandruff, and dryness.

How to use TTO to Heal Dry and Itchy Hair

Using your carrier, (olive oil, Jojoba, almond, or sesame oil) add at least two droplets of TTO to half a cup of your carrier oil. It is advisable to use little quantity of TTO if your hair is naturally oily, and a higher quantity if your hair is naturally dry. Warm your oil mix. Heat normal water on the stove. Before the water boils, remove the pot from the stove and set your oil in a separate vessel. Put your oil into the warm water until the oil becomes warm. Pour the oil on your wrist in order to feel the temperature of the oil so that it is not excessively hot. Divide the oil into 4 sections for easy distribution of the oil. You can make use of an applicator to apply the oil to all parts of your hair. Massage the oil mix into your hair scalp carefully. Now, cover your hair using a plastic shower cap and allow it for 30 minutes.

Head Lice Treatment

Tea Tree oil has been shown through various studies to destroy lice that are in their nymph and adult phases of life. It also decreases the number of eggs hatched by lice. Research also shows that ¼ children that were treated using chemical anti lice shampoo that contains pyrethrins and piperonyl butoxide were later free of lice. On the other hand, almost all the children that were treated with TTO were completely free from lice. The TTO can easily dissolve the sticky texture that links the nits to the shaft of your hair.

How to Use TTO to treat Head Lice

In a moderate bowl, combine 3 -4 droplets of shampoo and 3-4 droplets of lavender essential oil and mix it very well. Then add a quarter shampoo and mix it very well. Pour a little drop of extra virgin olive oil. This will help in suffocating the lice. Pour the shampoo mix into your hair and massage the scalp area very well. Put a shower cap on your hair and cover it for at least 30 minutes. Use your hands on your hair to remove the lice. Rinse it well. If you desire, you can apply hair conditioner for easy removal of the lice. Comb your hair so that the lice can be removed. Do this frequently for the next 7 days for all the nits, and the lice to be removed.

Tea Tree Oil for Skin

<u>Treatment of Acne with Tea Tree Oil</u>

Acne is a skin disorder characterized by black, red, or white pimples on the skin surface, particularly on the face of individuals suffering from it, which is caused largely due to the inflammation or sebaceous glands that are infected. This skin condition is common among adolescents. However, no matter how bad the acne may be, there is a good treatment that will heal acne completely through the use of Tea tree oil. As we have stated before, that TTO has antibacterial elements which help in dealing with acne. A simple 5 percent solution of TTO performs just like the majority of the popular acne drugs such as benzoyl peroxide.

<u>How to Use TTO in Treating Acne</u>

Dilute a little drop of Tea Tree Oil with about 20 - 40 droplets of witch hazel. Apply it to the skin surface once or twice daily using a cotton swab. You should do this cautiously as excessive use of TTO can dry your skin and make your own body to produce its oil which will make your acne worse.

Treatment for Eczema and Psoriasis

This is one of the great functions performed by TTO. It can be used for the treatment of Psoriasis and eczema.

How to use TTO to Treat Eczema and psoriasis

Mix a teaspoon of coconut oil and five droplets of TTO and another five droplets of lavender oil to produce a home-made TTO eczema lotion or any body soap.

Treatment of Minor Cuts and Infections

Tea Tree oil can also be used to treat minor cut and infections when it is mixed with lavender oil. It advisable to thoroughly clean the cut or infection with hydrogen peroxide or water. Then apply the TTO and properly cover the infection or cut.

Treat Ringworm

Tea Tree oil, being antifungal in nature can easily treat ringworm.

Before usage, you have to wash the area that is affected by the ringworm very well. To prevent contamination, any clothing that you use to dry the affected place must be put in the washing machine.

How to use TTO for Ringworm Treatment.

Sterilize your cotton swab and then add some few drops of oil to the end of the cotton swab. After that, apply the swab to the affected places. Perform this procedure three times daily for maximum results.

Removal of Makeup

You can use TTO to remove makeup from your face. To use it, get canola oil of a least ¼ cup and mix it with 10 drops of TTO in a 4 ounce glass jar that has been sterilized and shake it so that it mixes very well. Store it in a cold, dry place for use.

Treatment of Cold sores and Zap boils

If you want to use TTO to treat cold sores and zap boils, apply it directly to the cold sore. This should be done at least three to four times every day. Tea Tree oil can be used to treat staph infection, especially those have proven resistant to many antibiotic.

Soothes Athletes Foot

Tea Tree oil has been shown to treat athlete foot from burning, sealing, inflammation, and itching. If you are an athlete and you feel any of the above listed conditions, TTO can serve as a good means of treatment.

Effective Means of Controlling Gland that produces Skin Oil

Over production of sebum is one of the main causes of acne and dandruff. One of the main works that TTO does is to control skin oil production. Once it controls skin oil production, acne and dandruff will be prevented.

Treatment of Stye

Tea Tree Oil can be used to treat a stye, an inflamed swelling that occurs at the edge of the eyelid. A stye is often caused by bacterial infection. Since TTO possesses anti-bacterial properties, it is a good means of treatment. What the oil does is to decrease inflammation and bacterial activity.

How to use TTO to Treat Stye

Mix one teaspoon of TTO and 2 teaspoonfuls of water. The water should be properly filtered. Mix the two together and store it in a refrigerator. Carefully apply it around the eye three times each day until the pain, and the swelling disappears.

Treating Belly Buttons Related Infections

We have stated earlier that TTO has antibacterial and fungi elements. As a result of these properties, TTO can serve as a good treatment for belly buttons infections.

How to use Tea Tree Oil for the Treatment of Belly Button Infections

Mix 4-5 droplets of TTO with a teaspoon of olive oil or coconut oil. Use a neat cotton ball and gently apply the oil to the affected place. Allow it for 10 minutes and thereafter clean it off using a neat tissue. Do this for about three times each day until you begin to see results?

Healing of Dry Socket Pains

Dry socket pains, mostly experienced by individuals whose teeth have been removed can be treated with TTO due to its antiseptic properties. This can also be used to prevent tooth infection.

How to use TTO to Heal/Dry socket pains

Add two droplets of melt swab. Apply it to the affected place and let it remain for 5 minutes. Remove the cotton swap and rinse it with warm water. Carry out this procedure for 2 to 3 times every day.

Heal Blisters

You can use TTO to treat blisters.

Mix your TTO with plain or vegetable oil. Use a neat cotton ball and apply it to the affected place. It should stay for about 10 minutes before rinsing it with cold water.

Effective control of Body odor

If you are suffering from armpit odor, TTO can be used to control it owing to the presence of antibacterial properties. Since sweat does not smell, but rather the combination with bacterial that cause it to smell, then the antibacterial in TTO can serve as a deodorant and effectively control arm pit odour.

How to Prepare and Use TTO to Control Body Odour

Ingredients

3 tablespoons of coconut oil

3 tablespoons of shea butter

¼ cup of cornstarch

¼ cup of baking soda

About 20-30 Droplets of Tea Tree oil

Instruction

Melt coconut oil, shea butter in a moderate glass jar. Remove jar from heat when it has melted and pour in cornstarch, TTO, and baking soda. Wait for several hours for the mixture to be ready. Once it is ready, pour it into container/deodorant stick for use.

Use your finger to rub it under your armpit like a lotion.

Use as Diffuser and Room Spray

Tea tree oil can be used as air spray for the purpose of disinfecting rooms and nontoxic spay for removing bacteria and mold in the environment.

How to use Tea Tree oil as Room Spray
What you need:

4 Drops of Tea Tree oil

4 drops of Peppermint essential oil

4 Drops of lemon essential oil

4 drops of Eucalyptus essential oil

Now, mix all these oils before you combine them in a 2 ml glass bottle and roll bottle in between your hands for proper blending.

CHAPTER SIX

You Can Make TTO At Home

If you don't want to purchase tea tree oil from online, you can make your own tea tree oil.

Ingredients

A Bunch of tea tree leaves

Instructions

Pour a bunch of tea tree leaves in a pot. Cover the leaves with water. Set your vegetable steamer in a pot. Insert measuring cup in the steamer.

Cover the pot. Let the knob nub of your cover points in the direction of your measuring cup. Boil the water so that you can steam the leaves. Allow water to condense and eventually evaporate. The condensation is necessary so that it will slide to the handle and into your measuring cup.

Put 4 ice cubes on the top of the overturned cover/lid for rapid condensation of the steam. When the ice melt, put off the heat.

Take off your lid and empty the ice cube water into your kitchen sink. Take off your glass measuring cup.

Pour the substance into your measuring cup into a separation funnel. Seal the top of your funnel and then shake it thoroughly.

Overturn your funnel and open for the purpose of releasing the pressure in it. When you do this, the oil will easily float on the top of the water.

Place a glass bottle under your stopcock and discharge the water. Pour your oil into a coloured glass bottle.

Repeat this procedure for about three times for extracting all the oil from the leaves.

CHAPTER SEVEN

Tips and Tricks for Using TTO
Tips 1#: Excessive Drops

Never use excessive droplets of Tea Tree Oil as only a few drops will be sufficient with your carrier. When using your shampoo or conditioner, add 10 drops of TTO for each ounce of shampoo. When TTO is excessively used, it can lead to weak hair and other hair damages.

Tips 2#: Tough Dandruff

The reason why we employ the use of tea tree oil is simple. There are certain types of difficult and tough dandruff that shampoo may not deal with. It requires other forms of tougher measures; Tea Tree oil is one of those tougher measures. So when shampoo fails, ensure that you add a few drops of TTO with your carrier and be sure to see dandruff vanish within the shortest possible time.

Tips 3#: No Limitation

Tea Tree oil can be used for any type of hair texture. So whether your hair is short, small, tough, or, soft TTO can still be used with amazing results for your hair.

Tips 4#: Diluting Tea Tree Oil

Tea Tree Oil is strong that is why it has to be dissolved into another hair carrier such as olive oil, coconut oil, jojoba oil, etc., prior to applying it to your hair scalp. Whenever TTO is applied without diluting, it can lead to irritation and cause itchiness or even dryness. The moment you noticed irritation, dryness or itchiness, stop using TTO.

Tips 5#: Product Tip

As a result of its multiple functions, many products have incorporated some percentages of TTO in their products such as hair conditioners and shampoo. It is only when you use it that you can know what works for you.

Dosages of Tea Tree Oil

There is a recommended dosage of Tea Tree Oil.

Dosage For Adult

Acne: 5% TTO gel applied every day.

Infected eyelashes: Scrub the eyelid every week with 50% TTO and combine it everyday scrubs of the affected eyelid with Tea Tree Shampoo or 10% TTO. It should be applied once/twice daily for approximately 3 to 5 minutes for 6 weeks.

Nail fungus: 100% TTO solution that should be applied twice every day for the period of 6 months.

Athlete's foot: 25%/50% TTO solution that should be applied two times daily for at least 1 month.

Children Dosage

Acne: 5% TTO gel applied every day.

Infected eyelashes: scrub the affected eyelid every week with 50% TTO and everyday eyelid massages using about 5% of tea tree ointment

Side effects of Tea Tree Oil

Toxicity

Tea Tree Oil is very toxic when consumed orally. Whenever the oil is applied orally, it can lead to serious complications.

Skin Irritation and swelling

Tea tree oil may result in skin swelling and irritation in certain people. The oil can lead to dryness and itchiness in some people.

Hormonal Problems

When you use tea tree oil on the skin surface of young boys that have not yet attained the age of puberty, it can cause hormone imbalance. There are cases where boys begin to develop breast because of the TTO.

Mouthwash problems

When using Tea tree oil to gargle or wash your mouth, you need to be careful because the strong substances in tea tree oil have been shown to cause serious injury to oversensitive membranes in the gullet.

How to Buy Tea Tree Oil Online

There are various places that you can purchase Tea Tree oil online, but the popular ones are:

Amazon.com

Walmart.com

www.ingramcontent.com/pod-product-compliance
Lightning Source LLC
Chambersburg PA
CBHW020620220526
45463CB00006B/2636